CONTENTS

INTRODUCTION

Overview of Hiatal Hernia

A **hiatal hernia** occurs when part of the stomach bulges through the diaphragm into the chest cavity. The diaphragm is the muscle that separates the chest from the abdomen and plays a crucial role in the digestive process by helping control the opening between the esophagus and the stomach. When the diaphragm weakens or loosens, part of the stomach can push up into the chest, causing discomfort and a range of symptoms.

Hiatal hernias are quite common, particularly in individuals over the age of 50, but they can occur at any age. Many people live with a hiatal hernia without realizing it, as the condition may not cause noticeable symptoms. However, when symptoms do occur, they often involve acid reflux, heartburn, and chest discomfort, all of which can be aggravated by certain foods and eating habits.

Understanding Symptoms and Impact on Digestion

The symptoms of a hiatal hernia vary, but they most commonly include:

- **Heartburn** or acid reflux: A burning sensation in the chest or throat, especially after eating.
- **Regurgitation**: The sensation of food or liquid coming back up into the mouth.
- **Chest pain**: A feeling of pressure or discomfort, which can sometimes mimic a heart attack.
- **Difficulty swallowing**: Feeling as though food is getting

stuck in the chest.

- **Bloating** and **burping**.

These symptoms occur because the hernia can interfere with the normal function of the lower esophageal sphincter (LES), a muscle that acts as a valve to prevent stomach contents from flowing back into the esophagus. When the LES is weakened, stomach acid can escape into the esophagus, causing irritation and inflammation.

The Importance of Diet in Managing Hiatal Hernia

While medical treatment and lifestyle changes can help manage a hiatal hernia, **diet** plays a critical role in alleviating symptoms and improving quality of life. Certain foods can trigger or worsen acid reflux and heartburn, making it essential to choose meals that soothe the digestive system and avoid irritants.

The food you eat can either support or hinder your digestion. By incorporating the right foods and avoiding triggers, you can reduce symptoms, improve digestion, and help heal your body from within. This cookbook is designed with this goal in mind: to provide delicious, **hiatal hernia-friendly recipes** that promote digestive harmony and bring relief.

The Goal of This Cookbook: Healing through Food

The purpose of *Digestive Harmony: Tasty Recipes for Hiatal Hernia Relief* is to offer an approachable, easy-to-follow guide that empowers you to manage your condition through the food you eat. In this book, you'll find:

- **Nutrient-dense recipes** that support digestive health and reduce symptoms of heartburn, reflux, and bloating.

- **Practical meal planning tips** to help you prepare meals that fit your lifestyle and dietary needs.

- **Detailed, step-by-step recipes** for both main courses and desserts that are gentle on the stomach without compromising on flavor.

- **Guidance on avoiding trigger foods** while still enjoying the pleasure of eating well-balanced, satisfying meals.

Each recipe has been specifically chosen to soothe and support your digestive system, using ingredients that are easy to digest, non-irritating, and beneficial for managing a hiatal hernia. By following the principles outlined in this book, you can make informed food choices that help improve your digestion, alleviate discomfort, and support long-term health.

In the following chapters, we will dive deeper into what hiatal hernia is, the foods that best support healing, and how a balanced diet can lead to lasting relief. Whether you're newly diagnosed or have been living with the condition for years, this book is designed to guide you toward digestive harmony and a more comfortable, healthy lifestyle.

CHAPTER 1: UNDERSTANDING HIATAL HERNIA

What is Hiatal Hernia?

A **hiatal hernia** occurs when a part of the stomach pushes up through the diaphragm into the chest cavity. The diaphragm is a large muscle that helps separate the chest from the abdomen and assists in breathing by contracting and expanding. It also has an important role in the digestive process by supporting the esophagus and the stomach's opening. At the base of the esophagus is a muscle called the **lower esophageal sphincter (LES)**, which acts like a valve to prevent stomach contents from flowing back into the esophagus.

When a person has a hiatal hernia, part of the stomach slips through an opening in the diaphragm called the **hiatus**. This opening is naturally designed to allow the esophagus to pass through, but in cases of a hernia, the stomach protrudes through it, often leading to a weakened LES. As a result, stomach acid and other digestive contents can flow back into the esophagus, causing **acid reflux** or **heartburn**.

Hiatal hernias are classified into two main types:

1. **Sliding Hiatal Hernia**: This is the most common type, where the stomach and the section of the esophagus that connects to it slide up and down through the hiatus. These hernias tend to come and go and may not

cause symptoms unless they become large.

2. **Paraesophageal Hiatal Hernia**: This type is less common but potentially more serious. In this case, part of the stomach pushes up through the hiatus and remains there, potentially causing a risk of the stomach twisting (gastric volvulus), which can lead to severe complications.

Common Causes of Hiatal Hernia

While the exact cause of a hiatal hernia may not always be clear, several factors can contribute to its development:

- **Aging**: As we age, the diaphragm weakens, and the opening (hiatus) can widen, allowing the stomach to slide up into the chest cavity.

- **Increased Pressure on the Abdomen**: Excessive pressure in the abdominal area can force the stomach upward. Common causes include:
  - **Obesity**: Carrying excess weight can increase pressure on the stomach.
  - **Pregnancy**: The growing uterus can put pressure on the abdomen and affect the diaphragm.
  - **Chronic coughing or sneezing**: Frequent or persistent coughing, sneezing, or straining can increase pressure on the abdominal area.
  - **Heavy lifting**: Regularly lifting heavy objects can stress the abdominal muscles.

- **Congenital Defects**: In some cases, a person may be born with a larger-than-normal hiatus, making them more prone to developing a hiatal hernia.

Risk Factors and Symptoms to Look Out For

Several factors can increase the likelihood of developing a hiatal hernia, including:

- **Age**: People over the age of 50 are more likely to develop a hiatal hernia, as the diaphragm naturally weakens over time.

- **Obesity**: Overweight individuals are at higher risk due to increased abdominal pressure.

- **Smoking**: Smoking can contribute to weakening the LES, which may exacerbate the symptoms of a hiatal hernia.

- **Family History**: If you have a family member with a hiatal hernia, your chances of developing one may increase.

The most common symptoms of a hiatal hernia are:

- **Heartburn**: A burning sensation in the chest, often after eating, especially when lying down or bending over.

- **Regurgitation**: The feeling of acid or food coming back into the mouth or throat, particularly when bending over or lying down.

- **Chest Pain**: Discomfort or pressure in the chest that may feel like a heart attack.

- **Difficulty Swallowing (Dysphagia)**: Food may feel like it is stuck in the throat or chest, making swallowing uncomfortable or difficult.

- **Bloating and Burping**: A feeling of fullness or bloating, especially after meals.

The Role of the Diaphragm in Digestive Health

The diaphragm is essential for maintaining proper digestive function. Its primary function in digestion is to help regulate the LES and prevent stomach acid from backing up into the esophagus. The diaphragm, through its normal contraction and relaxation during breathing, helps to keep the LES tightly closed, forming a barrier against acid reflux. When the diaphragm weakens or loosens due to aging, pressure, or other factors, this protective mechanism can fail, leading to reflux symptoms.

Additionally, the diaphragm's role in breathing means that it is also involved in helping to regulate pressure within the abdominal cavity. A weakened diaphragm might not perform its job well, leading to more pressure and a greater likelihood of the stomach pushing through the hiatus.

How Hiatal Hernia Affects Digestion and Your Health

Hiatal hernia can disrupt normal digestion by causing **gastroesophageal reflux disease (GERD)**. GERD occurs when stomach acid frequently leaks into the esophagus, causing inflammation and discomfort. The LES, when weakened by a hiatal hernia, cannot effectively keep acid in the stomach, leading to frequent acid reflux and the characteristic heartburn symptoms.

In the long term, untreated hiatal hernias and GERD can lead to complications like:

- **Esophagitis**: Inflammation of the esophagus, which may result in ulcers and bleeding.

- **Barrett's Esophagus**: A condition where the cells in the lower part of the esophagus change due to repeated acid exposure, which can increase the risk of esophageal cancer.

- **Difficulty Swallowing (Dysphagia)**: As the hernia enlarges, it may interfere with swallowing and cause a sensation of food getting stuck.

For many people, a hiatal hernia can be a manageable condition with proper diet, lifestyle changes, and medical management. In cases of large or complicated hernias, surgery may be necessary.

CHAPTER 2: MANAGING HIATAL HERNIA WITH DIET

Managing a **hiatal hernia** primarily involves lifestyle changes, and one of the most effective tools at your disposal is diet. By choosing foods that are gentle on your digestive system, you can minimize symptoms like acid reflux, heartburn, and bloating. In this chapter, we will explore how food can help alleviate the discomfort associated with a hiatal hernia and the essential dietary adjustments needed to manage your condition.

How Diet Can Help Alleviate Symptoms

A well-balanced, **hiatal hernia-friendly diet** helps by:

1. **Reducing Stomach Acid**: Certain foods can help keep stomach acid levels in check and prevent them from flowing back into the esophagus.

2. **Promoting Better Digestion**: Foods that are easy to digest put less strain on the digestive system, which can help reduce symptoms of bloating, gas, and discomfort.

3. **Strengthening the LES**: A healthy diet can support the function of the **lower esophageal sphincter (LES)**, the muscle that prevents acid from backing up into the esophagus.

4. **Managing Weight**: Maintaining a healthy weight can reduce the pressure on the stomach and diaphragm,

minimizing the risk of symptoms flaring up.

By incorporating certain foods into your diet, you can create an environment that promotes healing, reduces irritation, and provides lasting relief from hiatal hernia symptoms.

Foods to Avoid: What Triggers Heartburn and Acid Reflux?

Certain foods can trigger or worsen **acid reflux** and **heartburn**, making them best avoided if you have a hiatal hernia. These foods relax or irritate the LES, allowing stomach acid to flow back into the esophagus and cause discomfort. Common triggers include:

- **Spicy Foods**: Chili peppers, hot sauces, and dishes containing strong spices like cayenne or curry can irritate the esophagus and trigger reflux.

- **Acidic Foods**: Citrus fruits (oranges, lemons, grapefruits), tomatoes, and foods containing vinegar can increase acid production in the stomach.

- **Fried and Fatty Foods**: Fried foods, fatty meats, and rich, creamy dishes can slow digestion and relax the LES, making reflux more likely.

- **Caffeinated Beverages**: Coffee, tea, and sodas that contain caffeine can stimulate acid production and relax the LES, increasing the risk of reflux.

- **Chocolate**: Contains both caffeine and theobromine, which can relax the LES and worsen acid reflux.

- **Mint**: Peppermint and spearmint can relax the LES and trigger heartburn, especially after meals.

- **Carbonated Beverages**: Soda, sparkling water, and other carbonated drinks can cause bloating and increased pressure on the stomach, which can exacerbate reflux.

- **Onions and Garlic**: Raw onions and garlic can irritate the esophagus and may trigger reflux in some people.

Limiting or avoiding these foods can help prevent symptoms from worsening, leading to a more comfortable digestive experience.

Foods to Embrace: Gentle and Healing Ingredients

While certain foods can exacerbate symptoms, there are many that are gentle on the digestive system and help reduce inflammation. These foods can support the healing of the esophagus, aid digestion, and prevent acid reflux. Incorporate the following into your diet for optimal relief:

- **Oatmeal and Whole Grains**: Oats, brown rice, whole wheat bread, and barley are excellent sources of soluble fiber that help promote digestion and prevent acid reflux. These grains also act as a buffer for stomach acid.

- **Lean Proteins**: Skinless poultry, fish, and plant-based proteins such as tofu and legumes are easy to digest and won't trigger heartburn.

- **Non-Citrus Fruits**: Apples, pears, bananas, and melons are low-acid fruits that are gentle on the stomach and can help soothe irritation.

- **Vegetables**: Leafy greens like spinach, kale, and lettuce, as well as carrots, cucumbers, zucchini, and sweet potatoes, are all easy on the stomach and help to reduce acid reflux symptoms.

- **Healthy Fats**: Olive oil, avocados, and nuts provide heart-healthy fats that support digestion without triggering reflux.

- **Ginger**: Known for its anti-inflammatory properties, ginger can soothe the digestive tract and help prevent nausea or discomfort.

- **Herbs**: Basil, thyme, oregano, and dill are flavorful additions to meals that don't irritate the stomach or relax the LES.

These foods work together to promote overall digestive health, strengthen the LES, and help reduce acid production, making them perfect choices for managing a hiatal hernia.

The Importance of Smaller, Frequent Meals

Instead of consuming large meals, aim for **smaller, more frequent meals** throughout the day. Large meals put pressure on the stomach and diaphragm, which can push stomach contents into the esophagus, causing reflux. Eating smaller portions allows the stomach to empty more efficiently, reducing the likelihood of acid backflow. It also helps keep the LES functioning properly, preventing it from relaxing too much.

Meal tips:

- Eat 5-6 smaller meals each day instead of 2-3 large ones.
- Avoid eating within 3 hours before bed to reduce the risk of nighttime reflux.
- Chew food slowly and thoroughly to assist digestion.

Hydration and Its Role in Digestive Health

Staying well-hydrated is essential for maintaining good digestive health. Water helps break down food, making it easier to absorb nutrients, and it also aids in the proper functioning of the digestive system. It is important to drink water throughout the day to support overall digestive function and prevent dehydration, which can worsen symptoms.

However, avoid drinking large amounts of liquid with meals, as it can increase stomach pressure and lead to reflux. Instead, sip water between meals and limit fluid intake during meals to small amounts.

Portion Sizes and Eating Habits for Better Digestion

In addition to choosing the right foods, portion control is a key factor in managing hiatal hernia. Overeating can stretch the stomach, increase pressure, and cause acid to backflow into the esophagus. Here are a few tips for managing portion sizes and improving your eating habits:

- **Mindful Eating**: Slow down and pay attention to how much you're eating. Avoid eating too quickly or overstuffing your plate. Aim to feel satisfied, not overly full.

- **Balanced Meals**: Include a variety of food groups (protein, whole grains, vegetables) at each meal to ensure a balanced, nutrient-dense diet without overwhelming your digestive system.

- **Avoiding Late-Night Meals**: Eating late at night or just before bed can increase the likelihood of nighttime reflux. Aim to finish meals 2-3 hours before lying down.

Sample Day of Eating for Digestive Harmony

To make these guidelines easier to follow, here's an example of a day's worth of meals that can help you manage a hiatal hernia:

- **Breakfast**: Oatmeal with banana slices, a small handful of almonds, and a drizzle of honey.

- **Snack**: A pear and a small portion of low-fat yogurt.

- **Lunch**: Grilled chicken breast with quinoa and steamed broccoli.

- **Snack**: A handful of cucumber slices with a dollop of hummus.

- **Dinner**: Baked salmon with sweet potato and a side of steamed spinach.

- **Evening Snack**: A small bowl of non-fat, plain yogurt with a sprinkle of ground flaxseed.

This sample day is rich in gentle, easy-to-digest foods that help minimize acid reflux and support digestion.

CHAPTER 3: TYPES OF FOOD TO EAT FOR HIATAL HERNIA RELIEF

Managing a **hiatal hernia** effectively through diet relies on understanding which foods soothe the digestive system and promote healing. In this chapter, we will break down the types of foods that are gentle on your stomach, support digestion, and help alleviate symptoms such as acid reflux, bloating, and heartburn.

To maximize your well-being, it's essential to embrace foods that are easy to digest, anti-inflammatory, and low in acid. By making thoughtful choices at each meal, you can help reduce the discomfort caused by hiatal hernia and encourage digestive harmony.

Easy-to-Digest Proteins: Poultry, Fish, and Plant-Based Options

Proteins are an essential part of a healthy diet, but certain types of protein can be more easily digested and less likely to trigger reflux or irritation. Here's a breakdown of good protein sources for people with a hiatal hernia:

- **Lean Poultry**: Skinless chicken and turkey are excellent choices because they are low in fat and easy on the digestive system. Avoid fried or heavily spiced versions, as these can irritate the stomach.

- **Fish**: Fatty fish like salmon, trout, and sardines provide healthy omega-3 fatty acids that are anti-inflammatory and support digestive health. Fish is generally easier to digest than red meat, making it a great option for individuals with a hiatal hernia.

- **Eggs**: Eggs, especially egg whites, are a great source of protein that is soft on the stomach. They are easy to digest and versatile in cooking, whether scrambled, poached, or in an omelette.

- **Plant-Based Proteins**: Tofu, tempeh, lentils, and beans are all excellent sources of plant-based protein that can be added to your diet. Choose options that are low in fat and avoid preparing them with heavy spices or acidic ingredients.

These protein sources provide essential nutrients and are relatively easy to digest, making them ideal for supporting your body's needs without overwhelming your digestive system.

Soothing Vegetables: Best Options for Your Digestive Health

Vegetables are rich in vitamins, minerals, and fiber, but some can be difficult to digest or trigger reflux. For individuals with a hiatal hernia, it's important to focus on **low-acid, non-gassy vegetables** that support digestion. Here are some great vegetable choices:

- **Leafy Greens**: Spinach, kale, and lettuce are all easy on the stomach and packed with nutrients. These vegetables help soothe the digestive system without increasing stomach acid.

- **Carrots**: Rich in beta-carotene and fiber, carrots are gentle on the stomach and are a great source of vitamins and antioxidants. They can be eaten raw or cooked, but cooking them makes them even easier to digest.

- **Zucchini**: This mild, non-acidic vegetable is light on the stomach and can be roasted, steamed, or added to stir-fries and casseroles.

- **Sweet Potatoes**: A great source of fiber and potassium, sweet potatoes are easy to digest and can provide a satisfying, nutritious addition to any meal.

- **Cucumbers**: Known for their high water content, cucumbers help hydrate the body and are easy to digest. Their mild flavor makes them an excellent addition to salads and smoothies.

While vegetables are essential for a balanced diet, it's best to avoid those that are gas-producing, such as broccoli, cauliflower, and Brussels sprouts, as they can lead to bloating and discomfort.

Low-Acidity Fruits: Gentle on the Stomach

Fruits are an important part of a balanced diet, but certain fruits, especially citrus varieties, can trigger reflux symptoms. For individuals with a hiatal hernia, it's best to focus on **low-acid fruits** that won't irritate the digestive tract. Here are some options to include in your meals:

- **Bananas**: Bananas are alkaline in nature, which can help neutralize stomach acid and prevent reflux. They are also easy to digest and packed with potassium, which supports digestive function.

- **Apples**: Apples, especially non-acidic varieties such as Fuji or Gala, are gentle on the stomach. They provide soluble fiber, which helps keep the digestive system moving smoothly.

- **Pears**: Pears are mild in acidity and high in fiber, making them an excellent choice for promoting digestive health and preventing constipation.

- **Melons**: Watermelon, cantaloupe, and honeydew are all low-acid fruits that are hydrating and gentle on the stomach. They can help soothe the digestive system and are great for people prone to heartburn.

- **Papaya**: This tropical fruit contains enzymes that can aid digestion and reduce bloating. It's especially helpful for easing the digestive process after meals.

Avoid highly acidic fruits like oranges, grapefruits, and pineapples, as these can trigger heartburn or irritation in people with a hiatal hernia.

Whole Grains and Fiber: The Importance of Balanced Carbs

Whole grains are an important source of fiber, which promotes healthy digestion and can help regulate bowel movements. For individuals with a hiatal hernia, whole grains should be included in the diet as they provide slow-releasing energy and are easy to digest.

- **Oats**: Oats are a great source of soluble fiber, which helps absorb excess stomach acid and provides a soothing effect on the digestive system. Oatmeal is easy to prepare and can be flavored with non-acidic fruits like bananas or pears.

- **Brown Rice**: Unlike white rice, which is processed and lacks fiber, brown rice is a whole grain that provides essential nutrients and supports digestive health. It's also filling and gentle on the stomach.

- **Quinoa**: A high-protein whole grain, quinoa is also rich in fiber and antioxidants. It's a versatile grain that can be used as a base for salads, grain bowls, or side dishes.

- **Barley**: Barley is another whole grain that's rich in fiber and can help prevent constipation while promoting digestive health. It's mild in flavor and easy to prepare.

These whole grains provide essential nutrients while supporting the digestive process, making them perfect for managing a hiatal hernia.

Healthy Fats: Supporting Digestive Health

Fat is an essential macronutrient, but when consumed in excess or in the wrong form, it can slow down digestion and trigger reflux. Healthy fats, however, provide essential nutrients without causing discomfort. Here are some fats that are good for those with a hiatal hernia:

- **Olive Oil**: Olive oil is rich in monounsaturated fats, which are beneficial for heart health and digestion. It also has anti-inflammatory properties that can help reduce irritation in the digestive tract.

- **Avocados**: Avocados are nutrient-dense and packed with heart-healthy fats. Their creamy texture makes them easy to digest and soothing to the stomach. They are also high in fiber and potassium, both of which aid digestion.

- **Nuts and Seeds**: Almonds, walnuts, flaxseeds, and chia seeds provide healthy fats, fiber, and anti-inflammatory benefits. They can help maintain balanced digestion when eaten in moderation.

It's important to avoid trans fats and fried foods, as these can exacerbate symptoms of reflux and cause discomfort.

Flavorful Herbs and Spices: What's Safe and What to Avoid

Herbs and spices can make your meals more flavorful without causing digestive discomfort. However, some spicy seasonings can irritate the stomach, so it's important to choose mild, soothing options.

- **Safe Herbs**: Basil, oregano, thyme, parsley, and dill are all gentle on the stomach and can add great flavor to your meals. These herbs are anti-inflammatory and can aid digestion.

- **Spices to Use Cautiously**: Ginger and turmeric are both excellent choices for soothing the digestive system and reducing inflammation. These spices are not only safe but also have healing properties for those with a hiatal hernia.

- **Avoid Irritating Spices**: Hot spices like cayenne pepper, black pepper, chili powder, and mustard can irritate the digestive system and trigger reflux.

By focusing on mild, soothing herbs and spices, you can add flavor to your meals without causing discomfort.

CHAPTER 4: MEAL PREPARATION TIPS FOR DIGESTIVE HARMONY

Effective meal preparation is key to managing a hiatal hernia and reducing symptoms like acid reflux, heartburn, and bloating. In this chapter, we will explore cooking techniques and practical tips that make it easier to prepare meals that support your digestive health. By using the right ingredients and methods, you can create meals that are not only nourishing but also gentle on your stomach.

Cooking Methods That Help: Steaming, Baking, and Grilling

The way you prepare food is just as important as what you eat. Certain cooking methods can make food easier to digest, while others can increase the likelihood of reflux or discomfort. Here are some of the best cooking techniques for people with a hiatal hernia:

- **Steaming**: Steaming vegetables, grains, and proteins is one of the gentlest methods of cooking. It preserves the nutrients in food while making it soft and easy to digest. Steamed vegetables, such as zucchini, carrots, and spinach, retain their flavor without becoming heavy or greasy. Lean proteins like chicken, fish, or tofu also benefit from steaming, as it helps keep them moist and tender without adding excess fat.

- **Baking**: Baking is another cooking method that is gentle on the digestive system, especially when you use minimal fats. Baking lean proteins like fish or poultry with herbs and vegetables creates a healthy, flavorful meal. Opt for whole-grain baking recipes such as oat or almond flour-based breads or muffins, which are less likely to irritate the stomach compared to white flour options.

- **Grilling**: Grilling is a great option for meats and vegetables, as it allows excess fat to drip away while maintaining the flavor of the food. However, it's important to avoid charring or overcooking the food, as this can lead to the formation of compounds that may irritate the digestive system. Grilled chicken, fish, and vegetables like bell peppers and zucchini are all excellent options for a hiatal hernia-friendly meal.

- **Sautéing**: If you prefer to sauté food, opt for a small amount of healthy oil (such as olive oil) and cook over medium heat. This method works well for vegetables, lean meats, and tofu. Avoid high-heat sautéing with excessive oils or fats, as this can make the food greasy and harder to digest.

- **Slow Cooking**: Slow cooking is a fantastic way to prepare meals without adding excessive fat or spices. Stews, soups, and slow-cooked meats can be made in a crockpot or slow cooker, which allows flavors to meld over a longer period of time without adding heavy seasoning or oils. This method is particularly useful for making hearty, soothing meals that are gentle on the stomach.

How to Layer Flavors Without Irritating the Stomach

While avoiding spicy, acidic, or fried foods is key for a hiatal hernia diet, it doesn't mean you have to sacrifice flavor in your meals. Here are some ways to enhance the taste of your dishes without irritating the stomach:

- **Use Fresh Herbs**: Fresh herbs like basil, parsley, oregano, thyme, and rosemary can elevate the flavor of your meals without causing discomfort. Herbs are also packed with antioxidants and anti-inflammatory properties that support digestive health.

- **Incorporate Mild Spices**: Mild spices such as ginger, turmeric, cinnamon, and cumin can add warmth and complexity to your dishes. These spices are not only flavorful but also have anti-inflammatory and digestive benefits. For example, ginger can help reduce nausea and soothe the digestive tract.

- **Use Olive Oil and Avocado Oil**: Instead of heavy creams, butters, or oils, opt for heart-healthy fats like **olive oil** or **avocado oil** to add richness to your meals. These oils are gentle on the stomach and provide essential fatty acids that support overall digestive health.

- **Infuse Flavors with Stock or Broth**: Instead of using salty or spicy sauces, consider using homemade vegetable or chicken stock to flavor your soups, stews, and sauces. Broths are light and soothing, providing depth of flavor without irritation.

- **Lemon Zest or Lemon Juice (in moderation)**: While lemon juice can sometimes trigger reflux, a small amount of **lemon zest** or a light squeeze of lemon juice can brighten up your dishes without adding excessive acidity. Use it sparingly and pair it with foods that are naturally alkaline, like leafy greens and grains.

- **Fresh Garlic**: Garlic, when used in moderation and

cooked lightly, adds a mild, savory flavor without overwhelming the stomach. Avoid consuming raw garlic, as it can be too strong for those with a sensitive digestive system.

Making Cooking a Healing Process

Preparing meals that promote digestive health can be a therapeutic process. Here are some ways to make meal prep both enjoyable and beneficial for your health:

- **Practice Mindful Cooking**: Take time to savor the cooking process and pay attention to the ingredients you're using. Consider how each item contributes to your well-being and try to focus on the healing properties of your food. Mindful cooking helps connect you to your meal and reminds you of the positive effects it has on your health.

- **Batch Cooking and Freezing**: Meal prep is a great way to ensure you always have healthy, digestive-friendly meals on hand. Consider batch cooking dishes like soups, stews, or casseroles and freezing portions for later use. This can save time on busy days and ensure you have access to nutritious meals when needed.

- **Focus on Balance**: When preparing your meals, aim to create a balance of **lean proteins**, **whole grains**, and **vegetables**. This combination provides your body with essential nutrients while also keeping the meal gentle on the digestive system. Plan meals around these building blocks to ensure you are getting a well-rounded diet that supports digestive health.

- **Avoid Overcrowding the Stomach**: Instead of preparing large portions, focus on making meals that are lighter and more frequent. Eating smaller meals throughout the day is better for digestion and can help prevent symptoms like bloating and heartburn.

Stocking Your Pantry for Hiatal Hernia-Friendly Meals

Having a well-stocked pantry with the right ingredients is essential for making meal preparation easier. Here's a list of essential pantry staples for people with a hiatal hernia:

- **Whole Grains**: Oats, quinoa, brown rice, barley, and whole wheat pasta.

- **Proteins**: Canned tuna or salmon, lentils, beans, chickpeas, tofu, and lean poultry.

- **Healthy Fats**: Olive oil, avocado oil, coconut oil, and almond butter.

- **Vegetables**: Canned or frozen vegetables like spinach, peas, carrots, and green beans (in case fresh produce is not available).

- **Herbs and Spices**: Fresh or dried basil, thyme, oregano, parsley, cinnamon, turmeric, ginger, and cumin.

- **Non-Dairy Alternatives**: Almond milk, oat milk, or coconut milk for cooking and baking.

- **Low-Sodium Broths and Stocks**: Chicken, vegetable, or beef broth to add flavor to soups, stews, and sauces.

- **Nuts and Seeds**: Almonds, chia seeds, flaxseeds, and walnuts (use in moderation to avoid too much fat at once).

- **Fruits**: Apples, bananas, pears, and melons (fresh or dried).

By stocking your pantry with these ingredients, you'll be ready to create a variety of healthy, soothing meals that support your digestive health and prevent discomfort.

Preparing Meals Ahead of Time: Tips for Busy Days

When you have a busy schedule, it can be hard to prioritize meal preparation. However, planning ahead can make a significant difference in your ability to manage your hiatal hernia. Here are some tips for preparing meals in advance:

- **Batch Cook Grains**: Prepare large batches of quinoa, rice, or barley at the beginning of the week and store them in airtight containers. These can serve as the base for several meals.

- **Pre-Cut Vegetables**: Chop vegetables ahead of time and store them in the fridge. This makes it easier to throw together a quick stir-fry or roast vegetables when you're short on time.

- **Make Simple Snacks**: Prepare small, healthy snacks such as cut-up fruits, raw nuts, or plain yogurt to have on hand when you need a quick bite.

- **Utilize Leftovers**: Use leftovers creatively to avoid food waste. For example, leftover chicken can be used in salads, wraps, or soups.

By taking these steps, you can reduce the stress of cooking while ensuring you always have healthy, gentle meals available.

CHAPTER 5: TASTY RECIPES FOR HIATAL HERNIA RELIEF

In this chapter, we will explore carefully crafted recipes designed to help manage and alleviate the symptoms of a hiatal hernia. Each recipe has been selected for its ability to soothe the digestive system while providing essential nutrients and delicious flavors. From breakfast to dessert, these meals are gentle on the stomach, easy to prepare, and free from ingredients that trigger acid reflux, heartburn, or discomfort.

Breakfast Recipes

Starting your day with a nutritious, stomach-friendly breakfast can set the tone for a day of digestive harmony. These breakfast options are rich in fiber, protein, and gentle ingredients that are easy on the stomach.

1. **Gentle Oatmeal with Banana and Almond Milk**
   - **Ingredients:**
     - 1 cup rolled oats
     - 2 cups unsweetened almond milk
     - 1 ripe banana, sliced
     - 1 tbsp chia seeds
     - A drizzle of honey
   - **Instructions:** In a saucepan, bring the almond milk to a simmer. Add the oats and cook for 5-7

minutes until soft. Top with sliced banana, chia seeds, and a drizzle of honey. Serve warm.

2. **Avocado and Poached Eggs on Whole Wheat Toast**
   - **Ingredients**:
     - 2 slices whole wheat bread
     - 1 ripe avocado, mashed
     - 2 eggs, poached
     - Salt and pepper to taste
   - **Instructions**: Toast the whole wheat bread. Spread the mashed avocado on top. Place the poached eggs on the avocado toast and season with salt and pepper. Serve immediately.

3. **Smoothie Bowl with Berries and Ground Flaxseeds**
   - **Ingredients**:
     - 1 cup frozen mixed berries
     - 1/2 banana
     - 1/2 cup unsweetened almond milk
     - 1 tbsp ground flaxseeds
     - 1 tbsp honey (optional)
   - **Instructions**: Blend the frozen berries, banana, and almond milk until smooth. Pour into a bowl and top with ground flaxseeds and honey. Enjoy!

4. **Apple Cinnamon Quinoa Porridge**
   - **Ingredients**:
     - 1 cup quinoa, cooked
     - 1 apple, peeled and diced
     - 1 tsp cinnamon
     - 1 cup unsweetened almond milk
     - 1 tbsp maple syrup (optional)
   - **Instructions**: In a saucepan, combine cooked quinoa, almond milk, and diced apple. Cook on

medium heat for 5-7 minutes until the apple softens. Stir in cinnamon and maple syrup. Serve warm.

5. **Yogurt Parfait with Berries and Oats**
   - **Ingredients**:
     - 1 cup plain low-fat yogurt
     - 1/2 cup mixed berries
     - 1 tbsp rolled oats
     - 1 tsp honey (optional)
   - **Instructions**: Layer the yogurt, berries, and oats in a bowl or glass. Drizzle with honey and serve chilled.

6. **Zucchini and Egg Scramble**
   - **Ingredients**:
     - 2 eggs
     - 1/2 zucchini, finely chopped
     - 1 tbsp olive oil
     - Salt and pepper to taste
   - **Instructions**: Heat olive oil in a pan over medium heat. Add zucchini and sauté until softened. Crack eggs into the pan and scramble with zucchini. Season with salt and pepper. Serve immediately.

7. **Chia Pudding with Coconut Milk and Blueberries**
   - **Ingredients**:
     - 2 tbsp chia seeds
     - 1 cup coconut milk (unsweetened)
     - 1/2 cup blueberries
     - 1 tsp vanilla extract
   - **Instructions**: Mix chia seeds, coconut milk, and vanilla extract in a bowl. Refrigerate for at least 4 hours or overnight to let it thicken. Top with

fresh blueberries before serving.

Main Course Recipes

These main dishes are designed to be filling, easy to digest, and gentle on the stomach, making them perfect for managing hiatal hernia symptoms.

1. **Grilled Chicken with Steamed Vegetables and Quinoa**
   - **Ingredients**:
     - 1 chicken breast
     - 1 cup quinoa
     - 1 cup broccoli, steamed
     - 1 carrot, steamed
     - 1 tbsp olive oil
     - Salt and pepper to taste
   - **Instructions**: Grill the chicken breast until fully cooked. Meanwhile, cook quinoa according to package instructions. Steam the broccoli and carrot until tender. Serve the grilled chicken with quinoa and steamed vegetables.

2. **Baked Salmon with Sweet Potato and Spinach**
   - **Ingredients**:
     - 1 salmon fillet
     - 1 medium sweet potato, peeled and diced
     - 1 cup fresh spinach
     - 1 tbsp olive oil
     - Lemon juice (optional)
     - Salt and pepper to taste
   - **Instructions**: Preheat the oven to 375°F (190°C). Place the salmon on a baking sheet and drizzle with olive oil, salt, and pepper. Bake for 15-20 minutes until cooked through.

Meanwhile, roast the sweet potato cubes in the oven for 20 minutes. Sauté spinach in a pan with a little olive oil. Serve the salmon with roasted sweet potatoes and sautéed spinach.

3. **Stir-Fried Tofu with Brown Rice and Zucchini**
   - **Ingredients**:
     - 1 block firm tofu, cubed
     - 1 cup cooked brown rice
     - 1 zucchini, sliced
     - 1 tbsp olive oil
     - 1 tsp ginger (optional)
     - Soy sauce (low-sodium)
   - **Instructions**: Sauté the tofu in olive oil until crispy. Add zucchini and ginger and stir-fry for another 3-4 minutes. Serve with brown rice and a splash of soy sauce.

4. **Ground Turkey and Butternut Squash Stew**
   - **Ingredients**:
     - 1 lb ground turkey
     - 2 cups butternut squash, peeled and cubed
     - 1 cup low-sodium chicken broth
     - 1 onion, chopped
     - 1 tsp thyme
     - Salt and pepper to taste
   - **Instructions**: Brown the ground turkey in a large pot. Add the onion and sauté until soft. Add butternut squash, chicken broth, thyme, salt, and pepper. Simmer for 20-30 minutes until the squash is tender. Serve hot.

5. **Vegetable and Chicken Soup**
   - **Ingredients**:

- 1 chicken breast, cooked and shredded
        - 1 carrot, diced
        - 1 celery stalk, diced
        - 1 cup spinach
        - 4 cups low-sodium chicken broth
        - 1 tsp garlic powder
        - Salt and pepper to taste
    - **Instructions**: In a large pot, combine the chicken, carrots, celery, spinach, and chicken broth. Bring to a simmer and cook for 15-20 minutes. Season with garlic powder, salt, and pepper. Serve warm.

6. **Baked Cod with Roasted Vegetables**
    - **Ingredients**:
        - 2 cod fillets
        - 1 cup baby carrots, peeled
        - 1 zucchini, sliced
        - 1 tbsp olive oil
        - Salt and pepper to taste
    - **Instructions**: Preheat the oven to 375°F (190°C). Season the cod fillets with olive oil, salt, and pepper, and bake for 15-20 minutes. Meanwhile, roast the carrots and zucchini in the oven for 20 minutes. Serve the cod with roasted vegetables.

Snacks and Side Dishes

These light snacks and side dishes are perfect for keeping you satisfied between meals without overloading your digestive system.

1. **Cucumber and Avocado Salad with Olive Oil Dressing**
    - **Ingredients**:
        - 1 cucumber, sliced

- 1 avocado, diced
- 1 tbsp olive oil
- 1 tbsp lemon juice
- Salt and pepper to taste

- **Instructions**: Combine the cucumber and avocado in a bowl. Drizzle with olive oil and lemon juice, and season with salt and pepper. Toss to combine and serve immediately.

2. **Roasted Carrots with Lemon and Dill**
   - **Ingredients**:
     - 1 bunch of carrots, peeled and cut
     - 1 tbsp olive oil
     - 1 tsp dried dill
     - Juice of 1 lemon
     - Salt and pepper to taste
   - **Instructions**: Preheat the oven to 400°F (200°C). Toss the carrots with olive oil, dill, lemon juice, salt, and pepper. Roast for 20-25 minutes, until tender.

3. **Quinoa Salad with Steamed Broccoli and Olive Oil**
   - **Ingredients**:
     - 1 cup cooked quinoa
     - 1 cup steamed broccoli
     - 1 tbsp olive oil
     - 1 tbsp lemon juice
     - Salt and pepper to taste
   - **Instructions**: Combine the quinoa and steamed broccoli in a bowl. Drizzle with olive oil and lemon juice. Season with salt and pepper. Toss and serve warm.

Dessert Recipes

Even with a hiatal hernia, it's possible to enjoy delicious, soothing desserts that won't irritate your stomach. These recipes are light, low-acid, and made with ingredients that promote digestive health.

1. **Banana Almond Cake (Low Sugar)**
   - **Ingredients**:
     - 2 ripe bananas, mashed
     - 1 cup almond flour
     - 2 eggs
     - 1 tsp cinnamon
     - 1 tsp vanilla extract
     - 1 tbsp honey (optional)
   - **Instructions**: Preheat the oven to 350°F (175°C). Mix the mashed bananas, almond flour, eggs, cinnamon, vanilla extract, and honey until combined. Pour into a greased baking pan and bake for 20-25 minutes. Let cool before serving.

2. **Chia Pudding with Coconut Milk and Blueberries**
   - **Ingredients**:
     - 2 tbsp chia seeds
     - 1 cup coconut milk (unsweetened)
     - 1/2 cup blueberries
     - 1 tsp vanilla extract
   - **Instructions**: Mix chia seeds, coconut milk, and vanilla extract in a bowl. Refrigerate for at least 4 hours or overnight. Top with fresh blueberries before serving.

3. **Apple Cinnamon Oatmeal Bars**
   - **Ingredients**:
     - 1 cup rolled oats
     - 1/2 cup unsweetened applesauce

- 1/2 tsp cinnamon
- 1 egg
- 1/4 cup almond flour

- **Instructions**: Preheat the oven to 350°F (175°C). Mix all ingredients in a bowl and spread evenly in a greased baking pan. Bake for 25-30 minutes until firm and golden. Allow to cool before slicing.

CHAPTER 6: LIFESTYLE TIPS FOR MANAGING HIATAL HERNIA

In addition to dietary changes, making certain lifestyle adjustments can significantly improve your ability to manage **hiatal hernia** symptoms and reduce discomfort. This chapter focuses on key lifestyle habits that can promote better digestion, support your healing process, and help you live more comfortably with a hiatal hernia. By combining proper eating habits with mindful practices, you can enhance your overall well-being and minimize the impact of the condition.

The Importance of Posture and Sleeping Habits

Good posture and proper sleeping habits are crucial for managing a hiatal hernia. Both can influence the pressure on the stomach and the functioning of the **lower esophageal sphincter (LES)**, the muscle that keeps stomach acid from flowing back into the esophagus.

1. **Posture:**
   - **Stand and sit up straight**: Maintaining an upright posture helps prevent excess pressure on the stomach. When you slouch or lean forward, you may inadvertently push stomach contents into the esophagus, which can lead to acid reflux and other discomforts.
   - **Avoid bending over after meals**: Bending

over puts pressure on your stomach and may trigger reflux symptoms. If you need to pick something up, try to squat or kneel instead of bending at the waist.

- ◦ **Support your lower back**: If you're sitting for extended periods, ensure you have proper lumbar support to maintain a neutral spine. This reduces the likelihood of slumping and the associated digestive pressure.

2. **Sleeping Habits**:
   - ◦ **Elevate your head while sleeping**: If you experience nighttime reflux or heartburn, sleeping with your head elevated can help prevent stomach acid from flowing back into the esophagus. You can achieve this by using an adjustable bed or propping your head up with pillows. Aim to raise the head of your bed by 6-8 inches (15-20 cm).

   - ◦ **Sleep on your left side**: Studies suggest that sleeping on your left side can reduce reflux symptoms. This position may help keep stomach acid in the stomach and reduce the likelihood of it moving into the esophagus. Avoid sleeping on your right side, as it may worsen symptoms.

   - ◦ **Avoid lying down immediately after eating**: Wait at least 2-3 hours after a meal before lying down. Lying down on a full stomach increases the risk of reflux and heartburn, as the horizontal position makes it easier for stomach acid to move up the esophagus.

Stress Management Techniques for Better Digestion

Stress is a major factor that can exacerbate digestive issues, including those caused by hiatal hernia. Chronic stress can weaken the LES, increase stomach acid production, and slow down digestion, all of which can worsen symptoms.

1. **Practice Deep Breathing**: Taking slow, deep breaths can help relax the body and reduce stress. Deep breathing exercises can stimulate the vagus nerve, which is responsible for regulating the digestive system. A simple breathing exercise involves inhaling deeply for 4 counts, holding for 4 counts, and exhaling slowly for 4 counts. Try doing this for 5-10 minutes each day.

2. **Mindfulness and Meditation**: Mindfulness practices, such as meditation and body scans, can help reduce stress and promote a sense of calm. Taking time each day to sit quietly, focus on your breath, and be present in the moment can significantly improve your digestive health. Guided meditation apps or YouTube videos can be helpful for beginners.

3. **Yoga and Stretching**: Gentle yoga and stretching exercises can help relieve tension in the body, improve posture, and promote relaxation. Certain yoga poses, such as the **child's pose** or **cat-cow stretch**, can help release abdominal tension and support digestion. Try to incorporate 15-30 minutes of stretching or yoga into your daily routine.

4. **Progressive Muscle Relaxation**: This technique involves tensing and relaxing different muscle groups in the body to reduce physical tension and stress. Start at your feet and work your way up, tensing each muscle group for 5 seconds, then releasing the tension for 10 seconds. This can help calm the nervous system and improve digestive function.

Exercise and Physical Activity Recommendations

Exercise is another essential component of a healthy lifestyle, especially when managing a hiatal hernia. Regular physical activity can improve digestion, maintain a healthy weight, and reduce the pressure on the abdomen that can lead to reflux.

1. **Low-Impact Exercise**: Activities like walking, swimming, and cycling are excellent choices for individuals with a hiatal hernia. These exercises are gentle on the body and do not put excessive strain on the abdomen. Aim for at least 30 minutes of moderate activity most days of the week.

2. **Strength Training**: Light strength training exercises, such as bodyweight squats, lunges, or resistance band exercises, can help build muscle tone and improve posture. However, avoid heavy lifting or exercises that strain the abdominal muscles, as this can increase the risk of reflux symptoms.

3. **Avoid Intense Abdominal Exercises**: Crunches, sit-ups, or other exercises that target the abdominal muscles should be avoided, as they can increase pressure on the stomach and worsen symptoms. Instead, focus on exercises that improve core strength without straining the area, such as pelvic tilts or modified plank poses.

4. **Take Short Walks After Meals**: Taking a short, gentle walk after meals can aid digestion and prevent bloating or discomfort. Avoid strenuous activity immediately after eating, but a 10-15 minute walk can help stimulate the digestive system and reduce the risk of reflux.

When to Seek Medical Attention: Signs and Symptoms

While lifestyle changes and dietary adjustments can significantly help manage hiatal hernia symptoms, it is essential to recognize when medical attention is necessary. If you experience any of the following signs, it is important to seek medical help:

1. **Severe or persistent chest pain**: If you experience severe chest pain, especially if it feels like pressure or tightness, it could be a sign of a more serious issue, such as a heart attack. If chest pain is accompanied by shortness

of breath, nausea, or sweating, seek emergency medical care immediately.

2. **Difficulty swallowing (Dysphagia)**: If you have trouble swallowing food or liquids, or if you feel like food is getting stuck in your throat or chest, consult your healthcare provider. This could indicate an issue with the esophagus or LES that may require medical intervention.

3. **Unexplained weight loss**: If you are unintentionally losing weight without making changes to your diet or exercise habits, it could be a sign of a more serious underlying condition. Contact your healthcare provider for evaluation.

4. **Frequent or worsening reflux**: If your reflux symptoms are not improving with dietary changes, lifestyle modifications, or over-the-counter medications, it may be time to seek medical advice. Your doctor may recommend prescription medications or further tests to evaluate the condition.

5. **Vomiting blood or black stools**: These are signs of bleeding in the digestive tract and require immediate medical attention.

The Role of Medication and Surgery

While most people can manage their hiatal hernia symptoms through lifestyle and dietary changes, some individuals may require medication or surgery to manage their condition effectively.

- **Medications**: Your healthcare provider may prescribe **proton pump inhibitors (PPIs)** or **H2 blockers** to reduce stomach acid production and help alleviate reflux symptoms. **Antacids** may also be recommended for short-term relief. Always consult with your doctor before starting any medication to ensure it's appropriate for your condition.

- **Surgery**: In rare cases, surgery may be necessary to correct a large hiatal hernia or if symptoms are not controlled with other treatments. The most common procedure is called **fundoplication**, where the top of the stomach is wrapped around the lower esophagus to prevent acid reflux. Surgery is usually considered when other treatments have failed, or if the hernia is causing significant complications.

CHAPTER 7: CONCLUSION

In this final chapter, we will wrap up the key concepts covered throughout the book and offer guidance on how to maintain digestive harmony moving forward. Managing a **hiatal hernia** is a journey that requires consistency, mindfulness, and a focus on long-term health. By incorporating the dietary tips, meal prep strategies, and lifestyle habits shared in this book, you can find relief from symptoms, reduce the risk of complications, and lead a more comfortable, healthier life.

A Final Word on Healing and Maintaining Digestive Harmony

The path to managing a hiatal hernia begins with understanding your body and being proactive about your health. While a hiatal hernia is a chronic condition, many individuals can successfully manage their symptoms with the right combination of diet, lifestyle changes, and medical support. The key is to be patient with yourself and give your body the time and care it needs to heal.

By focusing on **digestive harmony**, you are taking an active role in improving your overall health. This means being mindful of what you eat, how you move, and how you care for your body. Making small but consistent changes can have a profound impact on how you feel day to day, helping you manage your symptoms, prevent flare-ups, and support long-term digestive health.

Key Takeaways for Managing Hiatal Hernia

- **Diet is Essential**: The food you eat plays a critical

role in managing hiatal hernia symptoms. By avoiding trigger foods such as spicy, fatty, or acidic ingredients and embracing soothing, easy-to-digest options, you can minimize discomfort and support your body's healing process.

- **Meal Timing and Portion Control**: Eating smaller, more frequent meals helps prevent pressure on the stomach, reducing the risk of reflux and heartburn. Avoid large meals, especially before bedtime, to give your digestive system time to process food properly.

- **Lifestyle Adjustments**: Posture, sleeping habits, and stress management are all essential elements in the management of hiatal hernia. Practicing good posture, elevating your head during sleep, and incorporating stress-reducing techniques like mindfulness and yoga can greatly improve your quality of life.

- **Regular Physical Activity**: Gentle, low-impact exercise can help maintain a healthy weight, improve digestion, and reduce the pressure on your abdomen. Activities like walking, swimming, and yoga can promote overall digestive health and reduce symptoms.

- **Be Mindful of When to Seek Medical Help**: While lifestyle and dietary changes can help manage most symptoms, it's important to recognize when medical intervention is necessary. Severe symptoms, difficulty swallowing, chest pain, or vomiting blood should be addressed immediately by a healthcare provider.

Empower Yourself with Knowledge and Self-Care

The journey to managing a hiatal hernia is unique to each individual. By adopting a mindset of self-care and learning to listen to your body, you empower yourself to take control of your health. It's important to stay informed and consult with your healthcare provider regularly to monitor your progress and ensure that you are on the right path.

Remember that the goal is not perfection but progress. Every small change you make—whether it's choosing a soothing food, managing stress better, or practicing mindful eating—contributes to your overall well-being. Over time, these adjustments will help create a foundation for digestive harmony, improving both your physical and emotional health.

Moving Forward: Building Long-Term Healthy Habits

To ensure lasting relief and optimal health, it's important to continue building healthy habits that promote digestive wellness. Here are some strategies to help you maintain digestive harmony long-term:

1. **Continue Educating Yourself**: Stay informed about your condition and seek out reliable sources of information to help guide your choices. Medical advice, dietary adjustments, and self-care strategies may evolve over time, so it's important to stay open to new insights and recommendations.

2. **Stay Consistent with Your Diet**: While it's okay to indulge occasionally, maintaining a diet that is largely centered around easy-to-digest, nutrient-dense foods will support your healing process. Keep your pantry stocked with digestive-friendly ingredients and try meal prepping to make healthy eating easier.

3. **Listen to Your Body**: Pay attention to how your body responds to different foods, activities, and stress levels. Keep a food and symptom journal if necessary to track which foods or behaviors trigger your symptoms and adjust accordingly.

4. **Seek Ongoing Support**: Whether it's from your healthcare provider, a registered dietitian, or a support group, having a strong support system can help you stay

motivated and provide guidance along the way. Don't hesitate to reach out when you need help or advice.

5. **Prioritize Self-Care**: Manage your overall health by prioritizing self-care practices that go beyond diet and exercise. Take time for relaxation, get adequate sleep, and nurture your mental and emotional health. The mind-body connection plays a huge role in digestive health, and caring for both is essential for overall well-being.

Encouragement for the Road Ahead

Managing a hiatal hernia doesn't have to mean giving up the things you love. With the right tools, knowledge, and commitment, you can continue to live a vibrant, active life. The strategies outlined in this book will help you achieve **digestive harmony**, reduce symptoms, and take control of your health.

Every small step you take toward healthier eating, improved lifestyle habits, and stress management will lead to long-term benefits. Trust the process, be patient with yourself, and know that your journey to managing a hiatal hernia is unique and entirely in your hands.

Resources and References

At this point in the book, you may be looking for further support and information. While this book offers comprehensive guidance, the following resources can provide additional insights into managing hiatal hernia and improving digestive health:

- **Medical Providers**: Always consult with a healthcare provider before making significant changes to your diet or lifestyle.

- **Registered Dietitians**: A dietitian specializing in gastrointestinal health can provide personalized nutrition plans to help manage your symptoms.

- **Support Groups**: Connecting with others who are

managing similar conditions can provide emotional support and practical tips for living with hiatal hernia.

- **Educational Websites**: Trusted websites like the **American College of Gastroenterology** (ACG) and **Gastroesophageal Reflux Disease (GERD) support groups** provide up-to-date information on managing acid reflux and related conditions.

www.ingramcontent.com/pod-product-compliance
Lightning Source LLC
Chambersburg PA
CBHW051713250726
48653CB00007B/3009